Contributors

S0-ANO-476

1. Why travel medicine?
Mike Townsend (Diploma in Travel Medicine)
General Practitioner, Expedition Organiser and Leader,
Cockermouth, Cumbria

2. Preparation: equipment
Angela Robertson (Diploma in Travel Medicine)
Occupational Health Nurse, Robens Centre, The Surrey Research
Park, Guildford, Surrey

3. Preparation: advice on health risks
Lucy Elphinstone (Diploma in Travel Medicine)
Surgeon Generals Department, Ministry of Defence, London

4. Immunoprophylaxis
Iain Inglis (MSc in Travel Medicine)
General Practitioner, Bewdley, Worcester

5. Malaria
Jane Chiodini (MSc in Travel Medicine)
Independent Travel Advisor, Biddenham, Beford

6. Fitness to Travel/In transit
David Shand (MSc in Travel Medicine)
Occupational Health Advisor, St Richards Hospital, Chichester, West
Sussex

7. Travellers with special needs
Kitty Smith (Diploma in Travel Medicine)
Clinical Research Director, DuPont Pharmaceuticals, Stevenage,
Herts

8. Accidents
Eleanor Wilson
Nurse Advisor in Travel Health, Scottish Centre for Infection and
Environmental Health, Glasgow

9. Illness in travellers
Ann Dunbar (Diploma in Travel Medicine)
General Practitioner, Gordon, Berwickshire

10. After return
Mike Jones
Associate Specialist in Infectious Diseases, Care for Mission, Duns,
Berwickshire

Contents

Travel trends

An increasing number of British residents now travel abroad (Fig. 1). More than 43 million trips were made by British residents during 1998. Approximately 36 million of those trips were within Europe or to North America. However, 4.5 million visits were also made to countries where there is a higher risk of illness (particularly from communicable diseases) such as Africa, South America, the Indian subcontinent, the Far East and some parts of eastern Europe.

One survey conducted during 1996 showed that approximately 80% of all British citizens had either travelled or lived abroad at some time in their lives. From 1991–1996, over half of all British citizens had been abroad and 16% had been to an area where vaccinations should have been considered before their departure (Fig. 2).

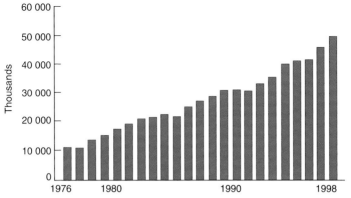

Fig. 1 Travellers overseas from Britain.

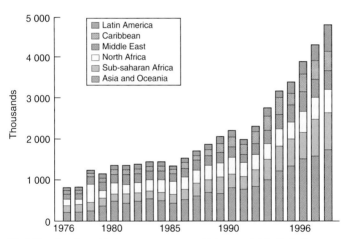

Fig. 2 Travellers from Britain to overseas areas with increased risk of infection.

Scope of travel medicine

The specialty of travel medicine has largely evolved in response to changing travel trends. Not only do many more people travel abroad, but the reasons for travel and types of travel have become much more diverse (Fig. 3). Whilst organised package tours remain popular, many travellers are becoming more adventurous and choose to backpack outwith 'tourist' areas, go on expeditions into remote areas sometimes in several countries or work as volunteers for prolonged periods. Travel for business purposes has become commonplace. In addition, potentially vulnerable groups of people such as the very young, the elderly, pregnant women and those with underlying medical problems or disabilities are travelling more than ever before (Fig. 4). As a result of these changes, more people need information, advice and in some instances, prophylaxis prior to or during travel.

Travel medicine is concerned with both the prevention and management of illness related to travel. Illness may result from exposure to infection but can also be caused by accidents, psychological upset, environmental hazard or political unrest. The specialty of travel medicine is therefore, a truly interdisciplinary and international specialty, involving numerous disciplines including, tropical medicine, infectious disease, microbiology, epidemiology and nursing, to name but a few.

Continued surveillance of illness and disease, both in the host country and in returning travellers, is necessary to allow sound risk assessments to be made for intending travellers. This is a crucial area for development within the specialty. Dissemination of information regarding real or potential risks can both prevent illness and increase detection of illness in travellers who have returned to their country of origin. This may have important public health implications when considering secondary cases or outbreaks as a result of travellers returning with infections.

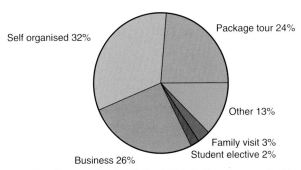

Fig. 3 Travellers attending Ruchill Travel Clinic in Glasgow categorised by reason for travel (n = 1596).

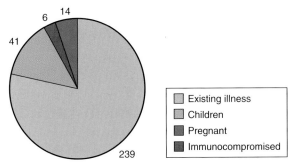

Fig. 4 Individuals with existing or special health problems out of 1596 travellers attending a travel clinic in Glasgow.

Points to consider when advising the traveller

A full 'risk assessment' should be carried out for every traveller.

Destination — What are the risks of diseases and other health hazards in the specific areas to be visited?

Mode of transport — Are there any potential hazards in the chosen method of travel, whether by air (Fig. 5), sea or overland?

Accommodation — Does the type of accommodation protect the traveller or expose them to potential risks (Fig. 6)? Are safety precautions and procedures in place or is there a risk of accidents, especially for the elderly or disabled.

Activities — The volunteer or business person may come into contact with the local population (Fig. 7). Those involved in sports or travelling in vehicles may be more prone to accidental injury. Holidaymakers and others who overindulge in alcohol may be more prone to expose themselves to sexually transmitted diseases.

Some travellers are more likely to have difficulties due to their age, lack of experience and underlying medical problems.

Refugees and migrants (those forced to migrate as a result of wars, famine or civil strife) are often more at risk of illness due to lack of access to essentials such as clean water, food, shelter and health care facilities, including immunisation.

Effect of travel on host countries

Travel and tourism has many benefits for the host countries but there are also drawbacks.

Traditional culture can be changed through exposure to foreign lifestyles. Local, essential industries may lose workers to more highly paid jobs in tourism with a migration from local communities to tourist areas. Crime may increase as poorer local people see the affluence of tourists. Sex tourism and use of recreational drugs and alcohol have greatly increased the spread of sexual and blood-borne diseases.

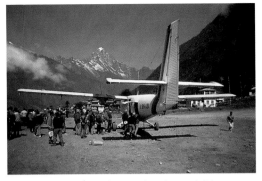

Fig. 5 Transport can vary between luxurious and risky.

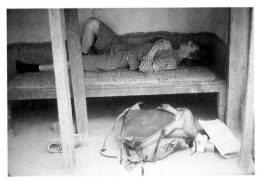

Fig. 6 Accommodation may be very basic and unhygenic.

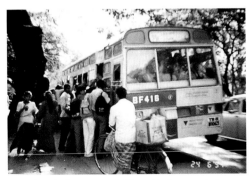

Fig. 7 A typically overcrowded bus aids the spread of respiratory disease.

Emerging and re-emerging diseases

Clear links have been seen between newly recognized diseases, re-emerging diseases, and their spread via travel.

Emerging diseases

The most notable example in recent years has been human immunodeficiency virus (HIV) infection and acquired immune deficiency syndrome (AIDS), which emerged in Africa and spread rapidly worldwide. The likely route was from Africa to the Caribbean, then on to the Americas, then Europe and Asia. The World Health Organization reported that it expected 29.4 million adults and children would be infected with HIV and that there would be 8.4 million cases of AIDS, by the end of 1996.

In 1991, cholera emerged as a major health risk in Peru and reached epidemic proportions.

Dengue is becoming an increasing threat in many areas including parts of Asia, the South Pacific and Central America, including the Caribbean—a popular tourist area (Fig. 8).

Malaria is seen increasingly in countries where it is not endemic, as a direct result of importation by travellers.

Re-emerging diseases

Diphtheria recently reappeared as a result of breakdown of vaccination policies in the former Soviet Union during its recent political upheaval, and this infection was then seen in neighbouring countries as it spread, again through travellers.

Tuberculosis has re-emerged in industrial and developing countries in association with poverty, drug resistance, overcrowding and AIDS (Fig. 9).

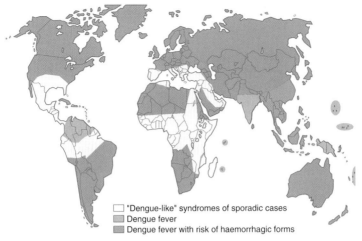

☐ "Dengue-like" syndromes of sporadic cases
▨ Dengue fever
▨ Dengue fever with risk of haemorrhagic forms

(Haemorrhagic form described in South America, mainly in Venezuela, since this date)

Fig. 8 Geographical distribution of dengue fever.

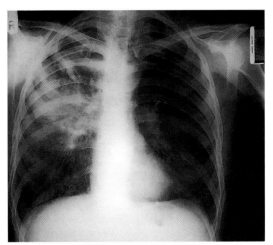

Fig. 9 Tuberculosis is an example of re-emerging infection.

Education and travel

Who has responsibility?

Health care professionals. Many doctors and nurses have received very little education in travel medicine. The need for education within the profession includes primary health care, occupational health and medical repatriation services.

Travelling public. Travellers have a responsibility to protect themselves; this includes attending for advice and prophylaxis, within a reasonable time scale, and taking precautions whilst abroad and sometimes on return.

Travel industry. It has been shown that the advice given by travel agents and holiday companies is often incomplete or inaccurate.

Key points to consider

- Reasons for travel include tourism, visiting friends and relatives, business, education, voluntary work, migration and displacement.
- Travellers may be exposed to jet lag, sunburn, cold, 'unsafe' roads, polluted water and contaminated food, and insect- and animal-borne diseases.
- Different or poor health facilities may include unfamiliar medicines, unsterile equipment and unscreened blood. Experiencing language difficulties during illness can be very stressful.
- On return home, counselling after exposure to illness and screening are often neglected—this may pose a threat to others who have not travelled.
- Travel medicine is concerned with emerging and re-emerging diseases such as AIDS, dengue fever, diphtheria, drug-resistant typhoid and tuberculosis as well as outbreaks of international importance including Ebola fever, plague, meningococcal infection and influenza.
- Modern electronic communications make surveillance more effective and allow access to up-to-date information (Fig. 10).
- Travel medicine is an interdisciplinary and international specialty.

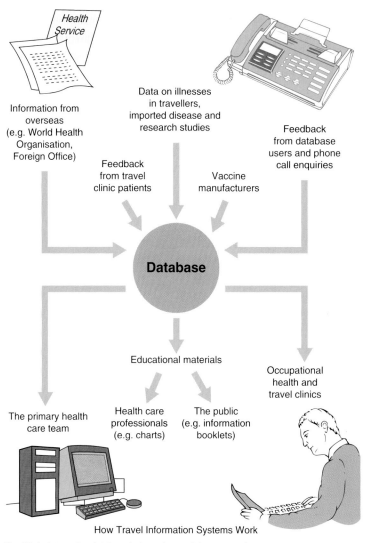

Health Service

Information from overseas (e.g. World Health Organisation, Foreign Office)

Data on illnesses in travellers, imported disease and research studies

Feedback from database users and phone call enquiries

Feedback from travel clinic patients

Vaccine manufacturers

Database

Educational materials

Occupational health and travel clinics

The primary health care team

Health care professionals (e.g. charts)

The public (e.g. information booklets)

How Travel Information Systems Work

Fig. 10 An interactive database helps to keep advisers up to date.

Documents (Fig. 11)

Passport

Passports should be correct and in date. Some countries require 6 months' remaining validity and may refuse entry if this is not observed. Children from Britain are now obliged to have their own passports.

Insurance

Adequate travel and health insurance is strongly recommended. Check carefully the level of medical cover and whether or not it includes repatriation to the home country.

Pre-existing medical conditions may not be covered if treatment is required abroad.

Pregnant travellers should ensure insurance includes any pregnancy-related treatment; some policies exclude claims arising from childbirth or pregnancy within 2 months of the estimated delivery date.

Hazardous activities such as jet skiing, parascending and hiring of motor bikes are almost certainly not covered by a general travel policy.

Immunisation

Yellow fever is the only internationally required certificate sanctioned by the WHO. Travellers may be required to produce an in-date certificate when entering or passing through some countries; they should check with their GP local travel clinic or immunisation centre at least 2 weeks before departure.

Visas

These may be required for entry to some countries.

HIV/AIDS test

May be required, especially for long-stay visitors. Check with the local travel clinic or host country embassy well before departure.

DoH T6 leaflet

Health Advice for Travellers in Britain contains useful information as well as an E111 form entitling travellers to reduced-cost emergency medical treatment in most European countries (Fig. 12).

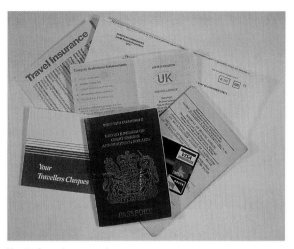

Fig. 11 Some important documents.

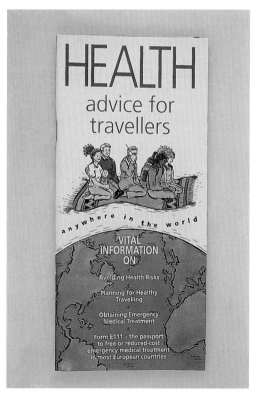

Fig. 12 Printed leaflets can reinforce verbal advice.

Mosquito nets

The use of close mesh mosquito nets may be necessary if travellers are sleeping in accommodation with unscreened windows or during camping/safari trips. They are available in single and double sizes and may be purchased from travel clinics and camping shops. They are light, compact and should be purchased before departure. Box 1 contains helpful tips on use of these nets.

Pre-treatment

For further protection, nets can be soaked in an insecticide solution of permethrin, dried and carefully re-packed in the original container to prevent damage during travel. The insecticide remains effective for 6 months provided nets are not washed.

Use

Suspend nets from hooks/poles when using indoors or tree branches outdoors (Fig. 13). Users, once inside the net, should ensure the net is securely tucked under the mattress or sleeping bag and that no mosquitoes are trapped inside.

Care

Ensure there are no tears in the net and inspect it regularly, especially if it is used outdoors.

Box 1 Tips on use of a mosquito net

- If not already impregnated, soak net in 10% permethrin solution before use
- Learn how to erect the net before departure
- Tuck net securely under the mattress—do not let it hang loose
- Inspect net regularly for tears

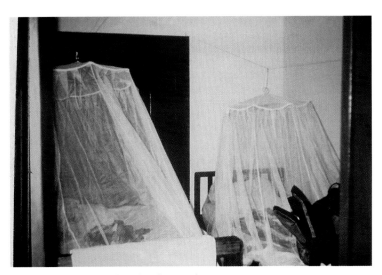

Fig. 13 Bell nets are portable and easily erected.

Safe water supplies

In urban areas, bottled water (preferably carbonated) is a feasible choice, but long-term travellers may need to find alternative methods of treating water.

Treatment

Aims are to remove solid particles (filtering) and kill harmful microbiological agents such as bacteria, viruses and cysts (purifying).

Filtration

A closely woven cloth or commercially produced filtration bag will remove sediment but not viruses or bacteria. Filtered water may require further treatment before it is safe to drink (Fig. 14).

Portable pump and gravity filters are available, which filter and purify the water, but care should be taken in choosing the most suitable apparatus.

Careful use and regular cleaning are essential to prevent contamination of equipment.

Purification

Boiling is the most effective method of sterilising small amounts of water but is not always the most practical. Water should be boiled for 1 full minute or 5 minutes at high altitude. Boiled water should be cool before drinking.

Chemical agents such as tincture of iodine 4 drops/litre (left to stand for 30 minutes) or chlorine tablets used according to manufacturer's instructions, may be used. It should be noted that these methods may not kill some cysts or viruses.

Storage

Treated water should be stored in sterile or disinfected containers covered with a lid; the container used for treatment is ideal.

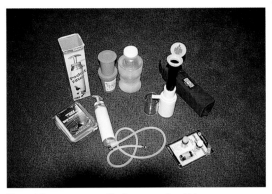

Fig. 14 There are many effective ways of purifying water.

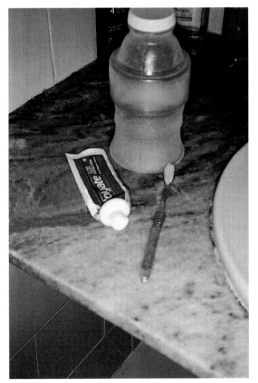

Fig. 15 Never forget that water used other than for drinking can cause infection, e.g. teeth cleaning.

Sun protection

The effects of sunlight are increased by the reflective properties of water and snow, and at high altitude (Fig. 16).

Sunscreens

These filter out the sun's harmful ultra violet radiation, mainly UVB/UVA rays and are available as lotions, creams or oils. The sun protection factor (SPF) number on the container indicates the length of time skin can be exposed to the sun before burning occurs.

An SPF of 12 delays burning for approximately 3 hours but should be used only as a rough guide. Box 2 provides a guide to avoiding sunburn including the use of sunscreens.

SPF numbers indicate protection against UVB rays whilst UVA protection may be indicated by a series of '••'

Types

Absorbent: these act by absorbing rays before they reach the skin. They are only effective against UVB rays, although some offer minimal protection against UVA rays. These sunscreens wash and rub off easily unless they are water resistant and require repeated application.

Reflectant: these are generally messier and thicker, and contain zinc oxide or titanium dioxide, which leave the skin looking white. They protect against both UVA and UVB rays and are good for delicate areas such as lips/nose.

Use

Apply before exposure to the sun and regularly during the day, especially after swimming/bathing or if heavy sweating occurs. An SPF of 15 or above is advisable for those with ordinary complexions and a higher SPF for those with delicate skin and for children.

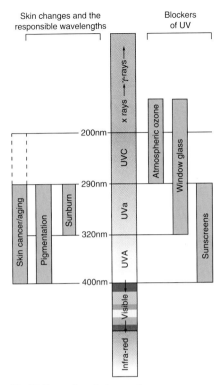

Fig. 16 The sun's emission spectrum.

Box 2 Tips on sunburn prevention

Acclimatise to the sun gradually with exposure reaching
  just 30 minutes a day
Apply sunscreens at least 30 minutes before exposure
  to the sun
Reapply sunscreens regularly, especially after swimming
Children and those with delicate skin should use
  sunscreens with a high SPF (15+)
Avoid sunbathing during the hottest part of the day
  (12:00–15:00 hours)

First aid supplies

Items for inclusion in a first aid kit depend on the associated risks of the impending travel (Box 3). Factors influencing choice may be location, duration of stay, type of accommodation, family members, access to medical facilities and current personal state of health.

Medications

All medications including an 'emergency' supply in case of loss, should be purchased before departure. Some may require a medical practitioner's prescription. Box 4 contains useful information on transporting and use of medicines whilst travelling.

General supplies

Aches and pains:
- soluble aspirin/paracetamol/ibuprofen.

Intestinal infections:
- broad-spectrum antibiotics (ciprofloxacin/ cotrimoxazole/metronidazole), particularly if visiting remote areas
- loperamide or lomotil
- commercial oral rehydration sachets or 'home-made' solution (Box 5)

Antimalarial tablets (if recommended)
- chloroquine/proguanil may be bought over the counter. Mefloquine and other antimalarials require a prescription.

Antihistamine/travel sickness:
- promethazine (may be used for either)
- terfenadine (antihistamine—prescription only)
- dramamine (travel sickness—over the counter).

Miscellaneous:
- calamine lotion (sunburn)
- oil of cloves (toothache)
- laxatives
- antifungal/antiseptic creams
- sleeping tablets
- personal, current medications
- insect repellent (spray/cream/wipes).

Extra supplies

Severe allergy:
- special adrenaline kit (food/bite/drug allergies).

Altitude sickness:
- acetazolamide
- nifedipine.

Box 3 First aid supplies

General items
- Adhesive plasters/tape
- Wound dressings
- Crepe/conforming/triangular bandages
- Safety pins
- Scissors
- Tweezers
- Antiseptic wipes
- Non-mercurial thermometers (individually wrapped paper ones are available, effective and easy to transport)
- Disposable gloves
- Small first aid booklet
- Torch
- Medications (see next section)
- Sanitary supplies (not always available abroad)
- Condoms (quality cannot be assured if purchased abroad).

Extra items
(For longer trips and visits to remote areas):
- Water purification tablets/equipment
- Sterile needle/syringe pack
- Emergency dental repair kit
- Hot/cold packs
- Insulating 'space' blanket

Box 4 Tips on carrying and using medicines whilst travelling

- Carry medicines in hand luggage to reduce the risk of loss
- Keep medicines in original labelled containers
- Absorption of antimalarials and contraceptive pills may be affected by diarrhoea and vomiting
- Extremes of heat/cold may affect efficacy of medicines

Box 5 Home-made oral rehydration solution

Dissolve:
- 1 level teaspoon salt
- 4 teaspoons sugar
in:
- 1 litre 'safe' water

Introduction

The majority of travel-related illness is not preventable by vaccination. Advice on prevention is essential and should be tailored to the individual and any particular risks he or she may face. A detailed travel history should cover:
- destination
- itinerary
- length of stay
- type and standard of accommodation
- activities (e.g. mountaineering, diving, aid work)
- an assessment of likely risk behaviour.

Behaviour

The traveller is at risk not just from the hazards of infection and adverse environmental factors, but also from his own behaviour. The consumption of alcohol may lead to a loss of inhibition and lack of compliance with preventive measures. Sunburn, accidents and sexually transmitted diseases (STDs) may result. Young people and other groups such as business travellers may be at particular risk of avoidable hazards when away from home. Education should be reinforced with written information.

Food- and water-borne infection

- Many diseases are transmitted by the faecal–oral route, usually via contaminated food or water.
- Only some of these infections (hepatitis A, typhoid and polio) are preventable by vaccine.
- For many other food- or water-borne diseases, the only preventive measure is careful attention to food and water hygiene.

Traveller's diarrhoea

- Affects up to 50% of travellers overseas.
- Frequently due to organisms such as *Escherichia coli*. A more severe and prolonged illness may be caused by *Shigella*, *Giardia* (Fig. 17), *Salmonella*, *V. cholerae* (Fig. 18) and *Campylobacter*.

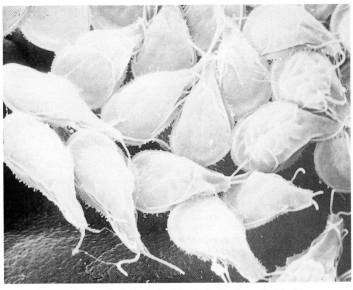

Fig. 17 Electron micrograph of *Giardia lamblia* attached to the wall of the jejunum.

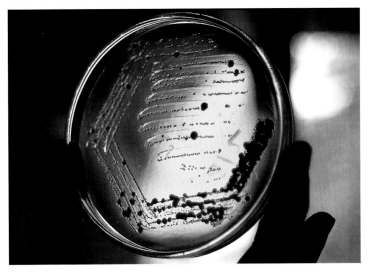

Fig. 18 *Vibrio cholerae* culture.

Advice on food and water hygiene

All travellers going outside north-western Europe, North America and Australia/New Zealand should be given the following advice:
- obtain purified water
- be selective in choice of food
- pay attention to basic principles of hygiene, such as regular hand washing.

Water

Outside developed, western countries tap water cannot be assumed to be of drinking quality.
- Bottled water, particularly if carbonated, may be used as an alternative, but in some countries this may also be of doubtful purity.
- Ideally, only well-known brands of bottled water with intact seals should be used.
- Alternatively, the traveller may purify water either by boiling or by using one of the many purification devices available.
- All water used for drinking, washing fruit and vegetables, and cleaning teeth should be of potable quality.
- Ice is often made from non-potable water and should be avoided.

High-risk foods

Foods considered healthy at home may be 'high risk' when travelling.
- Salads may not be washed, or worse, washed in water containing faecal effluent.
- Milk may not be pasteurised.
- Food is frequently left at high ambient temperatures for prolonged periods—beware of hotel buffets.
- 'Boil it, peel it or forget it' is a good rule of thumb in ensuring food is safe to eat. Travellers should choose fruits that they can peel themselves (Fig. 19).
- Food which is freshly cooked and served piping hot is less likely to transmit infection, such as hepatitis A (Fig. 20).
- Seafood may be a particular risk, not just from contamination with faecal organisms but from toxins, e.g. paralytic shellfish poisoning.
- In general, food served in good quality hotels and restaurants is likely to be safe, but it is still advisable to examine the menu and make a careful selection of low-risk foods.

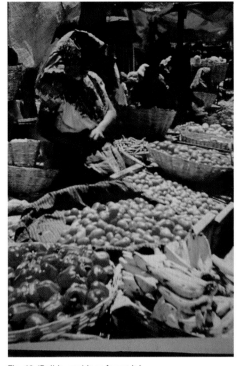

Fig. 19 'Boil it, peel it or forget it.'

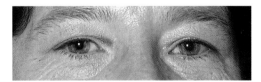

Fig. 20 Jaundice. Hepatitis A virus is spread by the faecal-oral route and is a risk with partially or uncooked food.

Insect-borne disease

A variety of diseases are transmitted by insects such as mosquitoes and other arthropods, e.g. ticks (Fig. 21). Malaria is the most well-known of these but there are many others, e.g. yellow fever and Japanese encephalitis. Some diseases cannot be prevented by vaccination or chemoprophylaxis, and are relatively common in the tropics, e.g. dengue fever and leishmaniasis. The problem may not be confined to the tropics, but present worldwide, e.g. tick-borne typhus (Fig. 22) and encephalitis in Europe, Lyme disease in Europe and the USA, Rocky Mountain spotted fever in the USA, equine encephalitis and Chagas' disease in South America, and a variety of mosquito-borne viral diseases in Australia. Travellers need relevant information regarding:

- type of insect vectors present
- time of day that is highest risk for bites
- seasonal variation in risk.

Advice should take into consideration the quality of accommodation, e.g. the availability of air conditioning and net-screened windows. Chemoprophylaxis to reduce the risk of malaria must always be supplemented with insect bite avoidance measures.

Disease transmitted by personal contact

Diseases of close contact

Tuberculosis, meningococcal meningitis (Fig. 23), and diphtheria are among the diseases that are more prevalent in developing countries and are spread by close contact, usually via respiratory droplets. These infections are more common in infants. The tourist is not at high risk, but those going for prolonged stays, or whose work brings them into close contact with the local population, should receive advice and, where appropriate, immunisation.

Sexually transmitted diseases

Tourists and business travellers may place themselves at risk of STDs through unprotected sexual intercourse. In many countries the prevalence of common STDs as well as HIV is very high, particularly among commercial sex workers. It is often difficult to identify the individual who might place themselves at risk in this way, and all travellers should be reminded of the dangers.

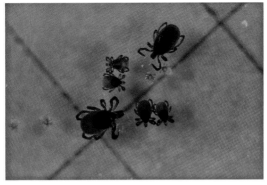

Fig. 21 Ticks can transmit a number of diseases.

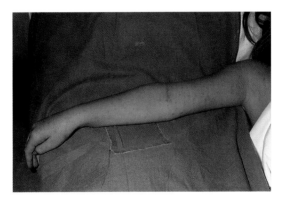

Fig. 22 The fine maculopapular rash of tick-borne typhus.

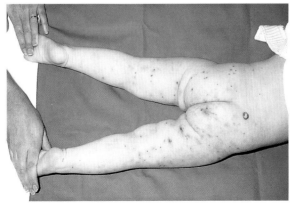

Fig. 23 The purpuric rash of meningococcal meningitis spread by the respiratory route.

Environmental risks

Travellers often worry about the risk of infectious disease but neglect to take precautions against the more common hazards presented by an unfamiliar environment.

Sun and heat

Sunburn is unpleasant and may increase the risk of skin malignancy, particularly in fair-skinned people. Exposure may provoke an attack of herpes (Fig. 24). Heat stroke is potentially life-threatening. Travellers should be advised to:

- prevent sunburn using high SPE creams
- limit time exposed to direct sunlight
- cover skin with loose, cool clothing
- increase their fluid intake, particularly if undertaking strenuous physical activities.

Cold

The risk of cold injury and hypothermia can be reduced by:

- wearing suitable clothing
- ensuring adequate food intake
- watching out for signs in each other by a 'buddy care' system.

Members of expeditions in cold climates should be suitably equipped and led by trained leaders.

Altitude and diving

Altitude sickness is a risk for all travellers going on mountain treks (Fig. 25). They require basic information on the early signs of altitude sickness (headache, sleep disturbance, anorexia), the need to acclimatise and the necessity to descend if symptoms persist or increase. Breathlessness and altered level of consciousness are late signs—often too late!

Diving may be risky for inexperienced individuals. Training and supervision is required. There is a risk of 'bends' on aircraft if dives are made within 24 hours of the flight home.

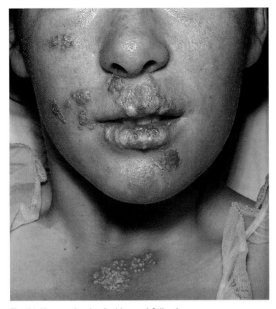

Fig. 24 Herpes simplex (cold sores) following sun exposure.

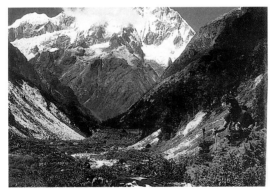

Fig. 25 Trekking and even skiing at attitude can lead to acute mountain sickness.

- Spiders, snakes and scorpions: travellers should take care when walking in undergrowth; they should wear boots and shake them out in the morning!
- Injury from sea urchin spines is very common— travellers should wear shoes when swimming in risk areas.
- Sea snakes and jellyfish in the sea may cause painful and sometimes life-threatening bites and stings—travellers should take local advice on safe places to swim.
- Hookworm larvae in damp sand or soil may enter through the skin and cause cutaneous larva migrans (Fig. 26)—travellers should wear shoes and avoid skin contact with soil or sand as far as possible.
- Schistosomiasis can be acquired by swimming or wading in infected fresh water (Fig. 27). The larval forms penetrate human skin and mucosa. They are present in Africa and less so in parts of South America and the Caribbean, the Middle East and south east Asia.

Rabies is endemic worldwide, the main exceptions being the UK, Scandinavia, Japan and Australasia. In the developing countries of Asia, Africa and South America, the principle reservoir is dogs. The disease can be transmitted by a bite, or by animal saliva in contact with mucous membranes or broken skin. Undue tameness in an animal may be an early sign of disease. All animals should be treated with caution and contact with stray animals, especially dogs, avoided.

Pre-exposure rabies vaccination is indicated for:
- travellers going to high-risk areas, particularly if remote
- long-stay expatriates
- animal-handlers.

All travellers, including those vaccinated, should be aware of the high risk from animal bites and the need for post-exposure vaccination.

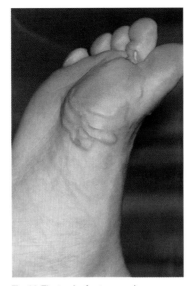

Fig. 26 The track of cutaneous larva migrans.

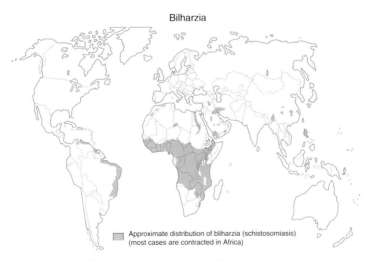

Bilharzia

Approximate distribution of bliharzia (schistosomiasis)
(most cases are contracted in Africa)

Fig. 27 Worldwide distribution map of schistosomiasis.

4 / Immunoprophylaxis

Introduction

Immunisation against infectious disease is an important tool to prevent illness in travellers and is one of the basic principles of preventative medicine. Vaccines clearly prevent only a minority of travel-related disease, but they are highly effective and very safe. Immunisations should be chosen for individual patients depending on the level of risk which they are likely to be exposed to.

Risk assessment

In advising a patient about immunisation, a thorough history must be taken to establish the likely exposure to particular disease hazards and the risk the patient may face in being vaccinated. It is important to avoid immunising where no, or minimal disease hazard exists or when patients have risk factors which make immunisation hazardous. The importance of an adequate patient history and a detailed description of the proposed travel arrangements are vital before an adequate assessment of risk can be made.

Patient-related factors

Current health and medical problems

The current health of a traveller is important. For example, immunisation is usually contraindicated where the patient has an acute febrile illness on the day of immunisation. Live vaccines are usually contraindicated where the patient is immunosuppressed due to diseases such as leukaemia and lymphoma. In these circumstances, inactivated vaccines such as the poliomyelitis vaccine (Fig. 28) are usually safe but possibly not as effective.

Pregnancy

Live vaccines should normally be avoided in pregnancy, although some such as yellow fever may be given after balancing the risks and benefits, if the risk of disease is high (Fig. 29). Measles, mumps, rubella, oral polio and BCG vaccines should be avoided. There is little evidence of risk during pregnancy with inactivated vaccines but most data sheets advise deferring immunisation if possible.

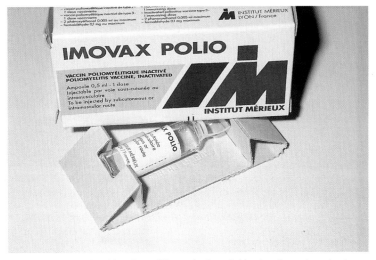

Fig. 28 Inactivated injectable poliomyelitis vaccine is available when live oral vaccine is contraindicated.

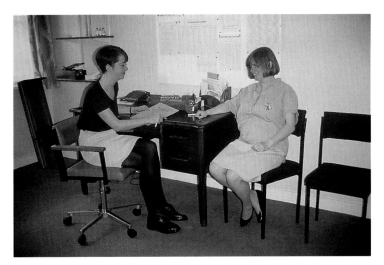

Fig. 29 Live vaccines should be avoided when possible in pregnancy.

Drug history	Recent chemotherapy or radiotherapy may have induced partial or complete immune suppression, which is a contraindication to live vaccines. Treatment with steroids may also have this effect, e.g. with prednisolone 60 mg/day for adults or 2 mg/kg/day for children for more than a week in the preceding 3 months. Chloroquine taken as malaria prophylaxis may inhibit the antibody response when rabies vaccine is given by the intradermal route.
Previous immunisation history	Immunisation status may obviate the need for primary courses but judgement on the need for boosters may be harder as many patients do not keep accurate records of previous immunisations. Prior immunisation with human normal immunoglobulin may reduce efficacy of live vaccines for 3 months with the exception of yellow fever.
Age	Many vaccines have lower age limits. This may either be due to lack of knowledge of effectiveness or safety in a given age group. Extremes of age in themselves are not contraindications to immunisation. For example, oral typhoid is contraindicated below the age of 6 years and Vi capsular polysaccharide typhoid vaccine is contraindicated below the age of 18 months, but rabies vaccine can be given at any age.
Sensitivities	Known severe reactions to previous doses of vaccines are contraindications to re-immunisation with the same vaccine (Fig. 30). An anaphylactic reactions to egg protein are a contraindication to egg-based yellow fever immunisation. Similarly very severe reactions to neomycin, penicillin or streptomycin are contraindications to oral polio and MMR immunisation.

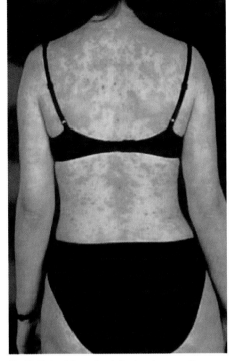

Fig. 30 Urticarial reaction following Japanese B encephalitis immunisation.

Journey-related factors

Destination(s)

This is one of the most important influences on planning an immunisation schedule due to differing patterns of disease endemicity in different parts of the world. Travellers to destinations in most developed countries should usually still be up to date with their polio and tetanus immunisations. To this must be added diphtheria if travelling to eastern Europe and especially the Ukraine and The Russian Federation. For travellers to the Third World, immunisation needs are much more variable.

Precise geography of area to be visited

This is important in that disease risks vary in different areas within specific countries. Figure 31 shows the areas of risk for meningococcal A and C.

Date of departure

This has an important influence on an immunisation schedule to ensure the vaccine will be at its most effective at the time of travel. Most primary vaccination courses take time (often 10–14 days) after completion to become fully effective.

Length of stay

The length of stay is important as risk can be directly related to length of exposure.

Season of travel

Season of travel can have an influence. For example, meningitis outbreaks in Africa occur generally during the dry season and Japanese B encephalitis outbreaks are more common during and following the monsoon months (Fig. 32).

Style of travel/activities planned

Visitors staying in good-quality hotels are much less likely to come into contact with disease than a backpacker living on a less than adequate diet, staying in poor-quality hostels or living rough. Adventurous activities may also increase risk by taking the traveller to more remote areas with poor access to medical facilities as well as increasing general level of risk due to the nature of the activities themselves.

Stopovers and diversions from planned schedule

Many travellers focus clearly on their final destination, particularly if they are planning a long journey and the risks from a short stopover may be overlooked. A very flexible plan may need an assessment of other risks to be catered for. Health professionals advising travellers must make specific enquiries in order to avoid these problems.

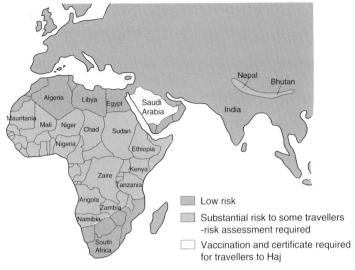

Fig. 31 Areas where meningococcal A epidemics occur.

Legend:
- Low risk
- Substantial risk to some travellers -risk assessment required
- Vaccination and certificate required for travellers to Haj

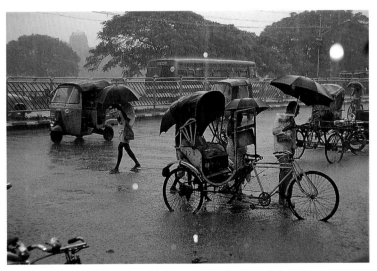

Fig. 32 Transmission risk can vary with the monsoon rains e.g. malaria and cholera may increase.

Vaccine administration

Cold chain

Must be maintained from despatch, during transit and on receipt.

Stock control

It is important to ensure that vaccines do not go out of date and that there are adequate supplies.

Clinic storage

Good storage must be ensured by keeping them in a refrigerator designed for vaccine storage, with a maximum–minimum thermometer and a log book kept up to date.

Guidelines

Clear and comprehensive protocols should exist for vaccine administration, storage and record keeping, especially where nurses take devolved responsibility from medical staff. These should be relevant and pertinent to the clinic and all individuals involved.

Record keeping

Adequate and consistent record keeping should be maintained.

Anaphylaxis

A rare but serious effect of vaccine administration. All who administer vaccines should be able to diagnose and manage anaphylaxis.

Diagnosis

Anaphylaxis is suggested when a patient has some or all of the following signs:
- pallor
- apnoea
- hypotension
- tachycardia (patients with syncope will have a bradycardia)
- wheeze
- angio-oedema
- cyanosis
- stridor
- urticaria.

Emergency equipment must be to hand (Fig. 33).

Management

- Place patient in the recovery position.
- Insert oro-pharyngeal airway and assist breathing if necessary.
- Summon additional help.
- Use adrenaline if necessary.
- Chlorpheniramine, hydrocortisone and salbutamol may all have additional roles.

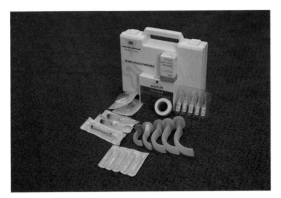

Fig. 33 Emergency equipment for management of anaphylaxis must be available where vaccines are administered.

Box 6 Sources of further information about vaccinations

Books
Useful for standard advice but need to be regularly updated. Examples include:
- *Immunisation Against Infectious Disease*, HMSO 1996 ('The Green Book')
- *British National Formulary* (BNF), BMJ Publishing – published regularly

Charts
These are free and useful for single journeys, but give limited geographical information and sometimes have conflicts of advice. Must be used in conjunction with other reference sources and the practitioner's own knowledge. Examples include: *Practice Nurse, Pulse, GP*

Examples of On-line and internet sources
Updated rapidly and are usually the most up-to-date sources. Perhaps will become the main source of current information but require a computer, modem and access to a telephone line.
- TRAVAX is available in the UK: http://www.travax.scot.nhs.uk (for professionals) or http://www.fitfortravel.scot.nhs.uk (for the public)
- Centers for Disease Surveillance in Atlanta, USA maintain an excellent site with up-to-date geographical recommendations and news of recent worldwide outbreaks of infection at: http://www.cdc.gov/travel/travel.html
- The International Society of Travel Medicine maintain a good general home page at: http://www.istm.org/ and have an especially good links page to several travel medicine sites worldwide at: http://www.istm.org/nonistm.html
- The World Health Organization has a large presence on the Web and the electronic format of their 'Yellow Book' is available at: http://jupiter.who.ch/programmes/emc/yellowbook/yb_home.htm
- Public Health Laboratory Service has an extensive Web site with information about emerging infectious risks worldwide as well as much information of general interest at: http://www.phls.co.uk/

5 / Malaria

Introduction	Malaria is caused by a protozoan, *Plasmodium*, transmitted to humans by the bite of an infected female *Anopheles* mosquito (Fig. 34). A total of 3–5 million cases of malaria occur annually, causing 1–2 million deaths. Transmission can also occur through blood transfusion and needle sharing in i.v. drug users, albeit rarely.
Clinical features	Malaria causes fever, chills, sweating and shivering. *Plasmodium falciparum* can cause: • jaundice • renal impairment • severe anaemia • pulmonary oedema • cerebral malaria (coma) • death. Most malaria deaths are due to *P. falciparum*.
The parasite	There are four different species of *Plasmodium*, giving rise to human malaria (Fig. 35): • *P. falciparum*. Occurs in almost all areas where there is malaria transmission. It is responsible for the majority of cases of malaria in subSaharan Africa, Haiti, the Dominican Republic, Amazon region of South America and parts of Asia and Oceania. This is the most serious form of malaria, responsible for most of the deaths, which occur primarily in children and pregnant women. • *P. vivax*. Transmission occurs throughout the malarious areas of the Americas, Asia, Middle East, North Africa, Ethiopia, Somalia and Sudan. • *P. ovale*. Found primarily in subSaharan Africa. • *P. malariae*. Transmission has a patchy distribution but occurs as a small proportion of the cases in all areas where malaria transmission occurs. For *P. vivax* and *P. ovale*, some of the sporozoites entering the liver become hypnozoites, dormant stages which develop to pre-erythrocytic schizonts at a much later date, sometimes 12–18 months later.

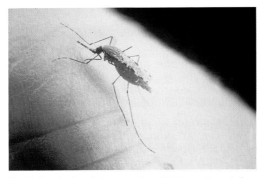

Fig. 34 Female *Anopheles* mosquito which transmits malaria.

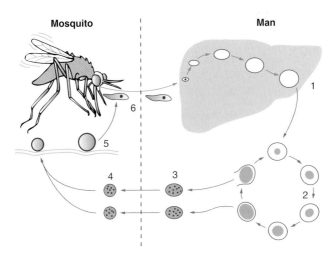

1. Merozoites develop from sporozoites in the human hepatocytes and are released into the blood.
2. Merozoites form trophozoites within the red blood cells (erythrocytes). They develop into schizonts, the red cells rupture and as merozoites the parasites are released into the plasma (this is when fever occurs).
3. Male and female gametocytes form in some erythrocytes to be ingested by the mosquito.
4. Sexual gametes develop in the mosquito and fertilisation takes place.
5. The resulting oocysts form in the mosquito stomach wall.
6. Mature oocysts rupture releasing sporozoites which migrate to the mosquito's salivary glands.

Fig. 35 Life cycle of the malaria parasite.

Prevention

There is no malaria vaccine available at present and prevention is based on four principles:

- **A**wareness of risk
- **B**ite prevention
- **C**ompliance with appropriate chemoprophylaxis
- **D**iagnosis and prompt treatment.

Awareness

The risk of contracting malaria not only varies depending on the part of the world being visited (Fig. 36), but also:

- area being visited (rural vs urban)
- length of stay/time of year (dry vs wet season)
- type of accommodation (air conditioned hotel vs camping tent)
- compliance with chemoprophylaxis
- bite prevention measures.

Pre-existing medical conditions, e.g. splenectomy or pregnancy can affect the severity of the illness.

Bite prevention

Mosquito bite prevention is as important as compliance with chemoprophylaxis. The *Anopheles* bite between dusk and dawn.

Prevention measures

Outside:

- If out after sunset, wear light coloured, long-sleeved clothing, long trousers and socks. Unprotected ankles are favourite sites for mosquito bites (Fig. 37).
- Apply insect repellent to exposed skin, preferably one containing over 10% DEET (n,n-diethyl-m-toluamide), or a eucalyptus oil base. Clothing can be treated with insect repellents. Always read manufacturer's recommendations.

In sleeping area:

- Air conditioning deters entry of mosquitoes.
- If room is screened, ensure windows and screens are shut before dusk and spray room with knockdown insecticide spray.
- Alternatively, sleep under a mosquito net, preferably impregnated with pyrethroids. Nets are available in cot to double bed size.
- Overnight, use electric pyrethroid mats indoors, or mosquito coils outdoors (Fig. 38).
- The use of electric buzzers, garlic and vitamin B is ineffective.

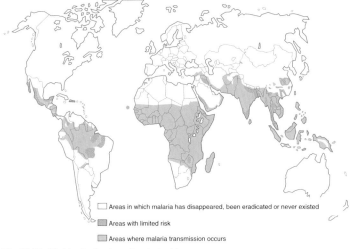

Areas in which malaria has disappeared, been eradicated or never existed

Areas with limited risk

Areas where malaria transmission occurs

Fig. 36 Worldwide distribution of malaria risk.

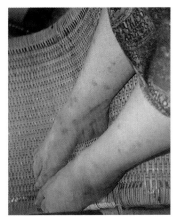

Fig. 37 Mosquito bites on unprotected ankles.

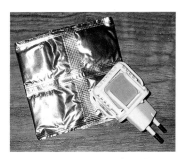

Fig. 38 Plug-in vaporisers are helpful in small enclosed areas.

Chemoprophylaxis

Malaria chemoprophylaxis substantially reduces the chance of getting malaria, and even if the person does get the disease, the chance of death is lower in those who take chemoprophylaxis.

The four most commonly used drugs for malaria chemoprophylaxis in the UK are chloroquine, proguanil, mefloquine and doxycycline. Proguanil is a causal prophylactic (acting on the pre-erythrocytic liver stages) and also acts on the asexual blood stages (suppressive prophylaxis). Chloroquine, mefloquine and doxycycline act as suppressive prophylactics.

Chemoprophylaxis should be started 1 week before entering the malarious area, except for mefloquine, which should be taken 2.5 weeks before to ensure tolerance and allow time to change if the traveller develops a reaction to the prophylaxis. The prophylaxis should be taken throughout the time in a malarious area and for 4 weeks afterwards. Compliance is vitally important. Appropriate regimens are defined by geographical area, taking account of the species of malaria parasite and likely extent of drug-resistant malaria present there. Underlying medical conditions may also influence the choice of drugs. Details are given in the malaria guidelines or the British National Formulary (BNF).

Diagnosis and prompt treatment

Breakthrough malaria should be diagnosed swiftly and treatment obtained promptly.

The minimum incubation period of malaria is 8 days. Most *P. falciparum* malaria causes illness within 3 months of being in a malarious area (Fig. 39). Presentation of *P. vivax* and *P. ovale* can be delayed due to the presence of hypnozoites.

The clinical features of malaria are non-specific and it is easily confused with other diseases, most dangerously influenza. It is *vital* that if travellers become unwell, they report their history of travel to a malarious area to the doctor or nurse.

Malaria cannot be reliably diagnosed clinically, so laboratory confirmation of the diagnosis is necessary. This is achieved by examination of thick and thin blood films (Fig. 40). New immunochromatographic strip tests are now available and are likely to be used widely.

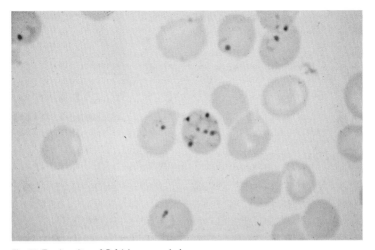

Fig. 39 Trophozoites of *P. falciparum* malaria.

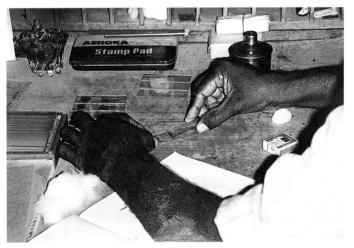

Fig. 40 Blood films being prepared for microscopy for malarial parasites.

Principles of treatment

If diagnosed early, malaria is easily cured (Fig. 41), but late cases of *P. falciparum*, with complications, carry a high mortality rate.

For some travellers likely to be remote from medical attention, standby treatment is advisable (Fig. 42).

Details of standby treatment regimens are given in the malaria guidelines or the BNF.

Conclusion

Malaria is a dangerous disease that is easily confused with other illnesses.

Advice

Sources of advice on malaria prevention may be obtained by the health professional from the following sources:

- Recorded advice for travellers from the PHLS Malaria Reference Laboratory is available on 0891 600350 (calls are charged by the minute).
- PHLS Communicable Disease Surveillance Centre (9 a.m.–12 md weekdays) London 020 8200 6868 ext. 3412
- Scottish Centre for Infection and Environmental Health (2–4 p.m. weekdays) for those who use the TRAVAX database (www.travax.scot.nhs.uk) Glasgow 0141 300 1130
- Hospital for Tropical Diseases—London 020 7530 3500 (treatment); 020 7388 9600 (travel prophylaxis)

Information can also be obtained by phoning:

London	020 7927 2437
Birmingham	0121 424 2000
Liverpool	0151 708 9393
Oxford	01865 225217 (personal answer)

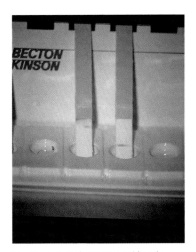

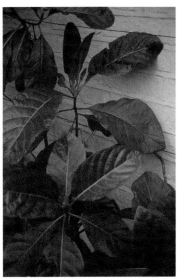

Fig. 41 Immunochromato-graphic strip tests may be useful for travellers using emergency self-treatment. The strip on the right is positive for *P. falciparum*.

Fig. 42 Quinine plant. Quinine is the original remedy for malaria and still very effective treatment for malignant disease. Other drugs are also available.

Introduction

The majority of health problems encountered by the traveller do not arise as a result of exposure to exotic infections but stem from pre-existing, perhaps latent, illness in the individual. The rigours and hazards of travel may, however, be implicated as a precipitating or exacerbating factor.

General

When advising the prospective traveller, as well as addressing issues such as malaria prevention and immuno-prophylaxis, it is important not to overlook pre-existing health problems. Amongst the common reasons for repatriation on medical grounds are medical diseases (in particular heart disease), surgical disease and psychiatric disorders. In-flight medical emergencies occur largely as a result of medical problems including cardiac arrest, unstable angina, exacerbation of chronic obstructive pulmonary disease and cerebrovascular accidents, although psychiatric problems also feature in this list.

There are few absolute contraindications to travel (Fig. 43) and even severely ill individuals can often travel with appropriate planning and support. However, if the lifestyle abroad or the journey itself is likely to aggravate pre-existing illness significantly, it may be appropriate to advise that the trip be cancelled. In this event, consideration of the reasons for travel will clearly be an important part of the decision-making process. More often advice will be centred on how to cope with the trip and what special arrangements may be needed.

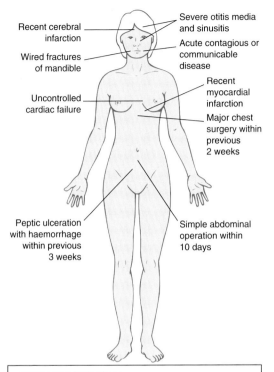

Recent cerebral infarction

Severe otitis media and sinusitis

Wired fractures of mandible

Acute contagious or communicable disease

Uncontrolled cardiac failure

Recent myocardial infarction

Major chest surgery within previous 2 weeks

Peptic ulceration with haemorrhage within previous 3 weeks

Simple abdominal operation within 10 days

Other contraindications
- Severe anaemia
- Contagious or repulsive skin diseases
- Pregnancies after 35th week(for long journeys) or 36th week (for short journeys)
- Introduction of air into body cavities within previous week
- Neonates (within first 2 days)
- Terminal illness
- Gross behavioural disturbances (e.g. serious drunkenness)

Fig. 43 Contraindications to flying.

Travel-related factors

There are few published guidelines on fitness standards for travel. Those that are available focus on conditions that are relatively common. For this reason the adviser should have an understanding of the potential hazards associated with travel, allowing a reasoned judgement to be formed where written guidance is not available.

Transit

Airport terminals, coach and railway stations can all be busy places where the traveller has to traverse long distances whilst carrying heavy luggage, all within a constrained time period (Fig. 44).

Prolonged immobility is common to all forms of travel over a long distance, and travel sickness, particularly at sea, is another frequent problem. Exercises can help alleviate circulation problems during these periods (Fig. 45).

Although many cruise ships have excellent medical facilities, whilst at sea, back-up is distant.

Cabin pressure within an aircraft is equivalent to that found at an altitude of 8000 ft. At this altitude, gas within the body can expand by up to 30% and the partial pressure of oxygen is reduced; this can present a risk to those with cardiorespiratory disease and other medical problems.

Destination

In developing countries, the provision of infrastructure, essential to public health, often lags behind tourism. Risks of contracting water and food-borne infections are therefore increased with the risk of de-stabilising underlying disease.

It is important to consider the effects of climate or altitude on any underlying medical condition, remembering that there may also be an unaccustomed increase in activity as well.

The need for access to adequate medical facilities should be considered. Cultural differences and language barriers can lead to difficulties when pre-existing health problems require monitoring, medication or treatment.

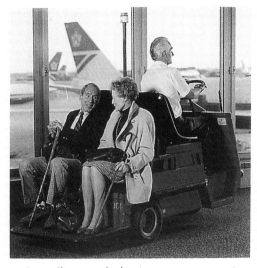

Fig. 44 Request assistance if necessary in airports.

1 Bring knees
to chest 5 times

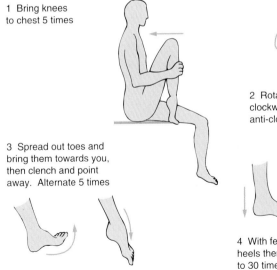

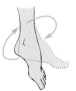

2 Rotate ankles 10 times
clockwise and 10 times
anti-clockwise

3 Spread out toes and
bring them towards you,
then clench and point
away. Alternate 5 times

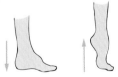

4 With feet on floor raise
heels then lower. Repeat 20
to 30 times

Fig. 45 Exercises to maintain circulation during long periods of immobility. (Courtesy of British Airways)

Specific problems (Fig. 46)

Circulatory disease

The stress of adapting to new surroundings may increase symptoms of ischaemic heart disease (IHD), heart failure and hypertension. Hot climates may aggravate postural hypotension resulting from the use of hypotensives, while diuretics can exacerbate salt loss.

Fitness to travel by air is an important consideration for the traveller with underlying heart disease. The reduced partial pressure of oxygen in the cabin at cruising altitude, may be enough to precipitate symptoms. Avoidance of alcohol and tobacco should be advised, as both may exacerbate hypoxaemia.

Patients who have been recently hospitalised due to IHD or congestive heart failure (CHF), are generally fit to travel by air if allowed sufficient space to move around. Those failing an exercise test will require supplemental oxygen during the flight.

Patients recovering from a stroke should not fly for the first 21 days.

The incidence of venous thrombosis and pulmonary embolus is increased by the prolonged immobility of travel. Patients with CHF belong to a high-risk group in this respect and aspirin prophylaxis should be considered.

A minority of pacemakers are interfered with by hand-held magnets used for security searches. Those who wear such devices should carry a letter warning of this risk.

Respiratory disease

Prospective travellers with pre-existing pulmonary disease may also be at risk from hypoxaemia during air travel. Patients who become breathless after walking 50 m on the flat need further assessment. If the PaO_2 during flight is likely to fall below 50 mm Hg, then supplementary oxygen is indicated. Even light exercise such as arm movement or walking in the aisle significantly increases oxygen demand, and the advice to remain seated contributes to immobility and its associated problems.

The response of asthma to changes in environment is unpredictable. Patients with stable asthma generally tolerate cabin hypoxia well, although air quality can be a problem. Bronchodilators should be close at hand.

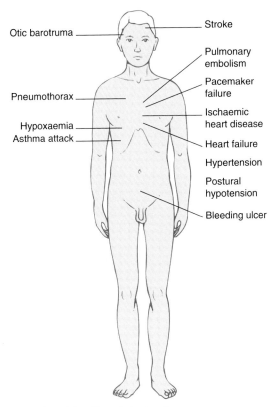

Otic barotruma

Pneumothorax

Hypoxaemia

Asthma attack

Stroke

Pulmonary embolism

Pacemaker failure

Ischaemic heart disease

Heart failure

Hypertension

Postural hypotension

Bleeding ulcer

Fig. 46 Potential problems during travel.

Diabetes	Diabetes is not a contraindication to travel but newly diagnosed, temporarily uncontrolled and 'brittle' diabetics should consider postponing travel until their condition is stabilised. It is important for diabetics to ensure they have adequate supplies of insulin, syringes and other equipment available in their hand luggage (Fig. 47).
	Unstable retinopathy is a contraindication to air travel as dilatation of retinal and choroidal vessels, in response to hypoxia, increases the risk of intraocular bleeding.
Gastroenterological conditions	Patients with active peptic ulceration should consider the availability of emergency surgery at their destination. They should not undertake a sea voyage of greater than 24 hours' duration. Following bleeding, a delay of 21 days is recommended prior to travel. Achlorhydria, secondary to medication or previous gastric surgery, predisposes to travellers' diarrhoea.
Surgery	Patients should not fly within 3 weeks of thoracic surgery, 1 week of intracranial surgery or within 10 days of abdominal surgery because trapped gas may expand and give rise to problems. Ventricular shunts are subject to stress with environmental change and should be checked for normal operation. Routine surgery, such as hernia repair and haemorrhoidectomy, is best attended to prior to prolonged trips abroad. Patients with jaws wired together should not travel unless quick-release fixings are in place or they are accompanied by someone trained to cut the wires.
ENT	Expansion of gas on ascent to altitude and contraction on subsequent descent can give rise to sinus and middle-ear problems. On ascent, gas escapes through the eustachian tube, but on descent it cannot pass back up the tube so readily. This may give rise to otic barotrauma, particularly with congestion caused by allergy or infection. There are various manoeuvres which may help equalise pressure and the use of a decongestant spray, prior to descent, can be helpful. After middle- or inner-ear surgery, air travel should be delayed for at least 2 weeks (Fig. 48).

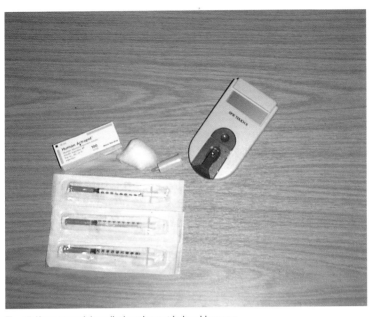

Fig. 47 Keep essential medical equipment in hand luggage.

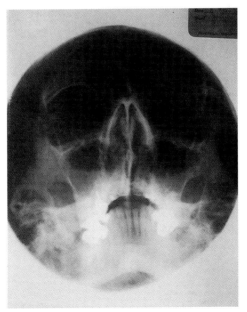

Fig. 48 Pressure alterations can be painful for sinusistis sufferers. Fluid levels can be seen in the maxillary sinuses.

Travellers suffering from epilepsy should be careful to ensure they maintain a regular sleep pattern as lack of sleep may increase the risk of seizure. If they suffer regular fits and are travelling unaccompanied, it is wise to inform airline crew of their wishes in the event of a seizure during travel.

- Patients with asplenism (functional or anatomic) are at particular risk of severe sepsis due to encapsulated meningococcus and haemophilus and should avoid travel to areas where risk of falciparum malaria transmission is high.
- Sickle-cell crisis is a risk for patients with sickle-cell anaemia when travelling above altitudes of 6000 ft. Air travel and high-altitude destinations are therefore hazardous to this group of individuals.
- Physical handicap is not a barrier to international travel but the need for careful anticipatory planning is vital. In particular, Third World countries have few, if any, facilities for disabled individuals.
- Blind travellers will experience difficulty if travelling unaccompanied (Fig. 49). Boarding instructions are usually made known via a visual display unit. Guide dogs cannot cross international boundaries without quarantine where required and canes may be removed from passengers during air travel.

Psychological and social adaptation

A psychological assessment is important prior to individuals' prolonged stays abroad (Box 7). Furthermore, travelling may be the first overt symptom of hypomania and rapid time zone changes can precipitate affective disorders in pre-disposed individuals. Serious psychiatric disorders, alcohol dependence or regular use of tranquillisers should all be viewed as possible contraindications to travel. Schizophrenics do not take changes of culture easily and a tendency to paranoia at home may be a contraindication to travel.

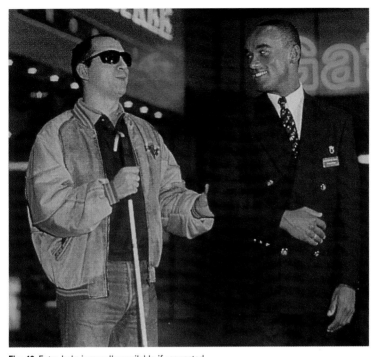

Fig. 49 Extra help is usually available if requested.

Box 7 Psychological contraindications to travel or work overseas

- Schizophrenia
- Bipolar or unipolar affective disorder
- Certain personality disorders
- Alcoholism or illicit drug use
- Chronic fatigue syndrome

Pre-travel assessment

It is important to consider the stability of any medical condition, the individual's fitness to cope with the hazards that can be expected, their emotional stability and the effect any complaint may have on fellow travellers. Airlines can refuse to carry passengers who may cause distress to other passengers. Infectious diseases, incontinence, psychiatric illness and severe skin complaints may all qualify in this respect.

A checklist for assessing a traveller's fitness to travel should include a review of their medical history and current treatment, physical examination and assessment of exercise tolerance (Fig. 50). Enquiry about previous travel experience may be helpful. Further assessment may be indicated, including an electrocardiogram (ECG), haemoglobin levels (and blood group for prolonged stays), a chest X-ray (if lung bullae or pneumothorax is suspected) and specialised lung function or cardiac stress testing. For prolonged stays, routine examinations such as dental, ophthalmic and well woman checks should be considered.

Planning

Patients with significant medical problems should carry a letter from a physician or alternatively a 'Medic Alert' bracelet can be worn. Consider what forms of care or treatment may be required abroad. The International Association for Medical Assistance to Travellers (IAMAT) provides lists of English-speaking doctors throughout the world. Special requirements such as wheelchairs, assistance with luggage or supplementary oxygen should be booked well in advance.

The International Air Transport Association has developed a standard medical information form (MEDIF). Frequent travellers with stable conditions can apply for a frequent flyer's medical card (FREMED) issued by airline medical departments. Many support groups (e.g. the British Diabetic Association) organise foreign excursions that are geared to take account of any special requirements.

EXAMPLE OF A FORM WHICH CAN BE USED TO MAKE RISK ASSESSMENTS

Name:	G.P:
Address:	Address:
D.O.B.	Unit Number

PATIENT DETAILS:

Medical History:	
Current illnesses:	
Current medication:	
Allergies:	Pregnancy:

TRAVEL DETAILS

Destination(s):	
Duration of stay:	Date of departure:

Type of trip

Package holiday	Business < 3 months Occupation:	Business > 3 months Occupation:
Self org. visit	Backpacking	Voluntary work
Visiting family	Elective	Other

Areas to be visited

Urban only	Urban and rural	Rural only	Altitude > 3000 m Describe:

Accommodation

Good	Basic	Poor

MALARIA

Bite avoidance discussed	Standby Treatment:

Prophylaxis advised

Chloroquine	Proguanil	Doxycycline	Mefloquine	Malarone	None	

Notes:

Fig. 50 A thorough pre-travel risk assessment is advised.

In transit

Motion sickness

Women and children between the ages of 3 and 12 years may be slightly more susceptible to motion sickness. Other predisposing factors influencing predisposition include alcohol, fatigue and sitting towards the rear of a vehicle. Symptoms may be eased or even allayed by limiting food and alcohol intake, sitting in the front seat of a vehicle and having a window open. Some travellers find wearing bands that apply pressure on a point above the wrist of some benefit. Drugs such as antihistamines, anticholinergics or tranquillisers may be given to prevent motion sickness but can cause drowsiness and should not be taken with alcohol.

Fear of flying

May be a problem for inexperienced or frequent air travellers. Some major airlines offer courses for passengers to assist in overcoming fear of flying. Mild sedatives, or alternative relaxation therapies may reduce the anxiety that flying may induce.

Jet lag

This is the result of an upset in the body's circadian rhythms, which is the normal pattern of sleep and activity affected by stimuli such as day and night, time and temperature. The change of these environmental factors when crossing several time zones means that some travellers may experience sleepiness during the day and alertness at night. Those taking eastward flights fare worse than those taking westward flights.

Air sickness

Air sickness is usually associated with severe turbulence during a flight. Steps can be taken to reduce the symptoms of motion sickness as mentioned previously and travellers may wish to consider sitting between the wings or towards the front of an aircraft.

Sea sickness

The incidence of sea sickness on large vessels has reduced with the introduction of ships' stabilisers. Steps to avoid motion sickness can be taken and sea passengers may benefit from lying down and keeping their heads still. Adaptation to rough seas usually occurs within a few days.

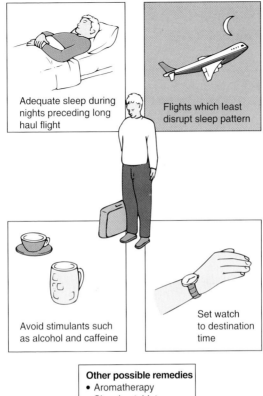

Adequate sleep during nights preceding long haul flight

Flights which least disrupt sleep pattern

Avoid stimulants such as alcohol and caffeine

Set watch to destination time

Other possible remedies
- Aromatherapy
- Sleeping tablets
- Modified diet
- Exercise
- Increased exposure to bright light
- Melatonin

Fig. 51 Steps to help minimise the effects of jet lag.

7 / Travellers with special needs

Introduction

Some groups of travellers may be at greater risk of travel-related health problems as a result of their medical, physiological, physical or psychological characteristics (Box 8). These travellers have special needs, either because they are more likely to suffer health problems while travelling or because if they do encounter such problems, the outcome is likely to be worse than for other groups of travellers. Their needs must be met if they are to travel safely.

Advising travellers with special needs

- The aim is to reduce the risk and/or severity of travel-related health problems
- The key is good pre-trip planning, started well before the date of departure.
- An accurate assessment of risk must be made. This requires a thorough knowledge of:
  1. Travel plans
  2. Medical history.

Medical history

Patients with the following conditions would be considered to have special needs.
- Pre-existing health problems, e.g. diabetes, angina
- History of travel-related health problems
- Physical disabilities
- Obstetric history of concern
- Current symptoms of concern
- Current pregnancy
- Management of existing problems
- History of psychological illness
- Current medication allergies.

Travel health issues for pregnant women

Travel health risks may affect the pregnant woman, the fetus or both (Box 9). Risk is related to:
- health of mother
- gestational age of fetus
- previous obstetric history.

Box 8 Travellers with special needs

- Pregnant women
- Babies and children
- Elderly travellers
- Disabled travellers
- Travellers with pre-existing medical conditions
- HIV-positive travellers

Box 9 Travel health issues for pregnant women

Immunisation
Risk/benefit must be carefully assessed before using any vaccine in pregnancy, especially in the first trimester. Live vaccines should be avoided.

Malaria prophylaxis
Malaria may be more severe in pregnancy. Prophylaxis must be safe for mother and fetus. Insect bites should be avoided when possible.

Medication
Drugs available over the counter (OTC) in some countries may be unsafe for use in pregnancy.

Flying
Most airlines do not allow pregnant women to fly after 36 weeks of pregnancy.

Medical care
Antenatal care may be interrupted. Access to good medical care may be limited and the standard of care lower than in the UK. There may be risk of poorly sterilised equipment and contaminated blood received through transfusion.

Insurance
Comprehensive insurance is vital—pregnant travellers should check for exclusions prior to departure. Insurance should cover emergency medical repatriation.

Babies and children

Diarrhoeal disease

Babies and small children are at higher risk of contracting pathogens via the faecal–oral route. They may become rapidly dehydrated when suffering from diarrhoea. Good hygiene should be enforced, including teaching children to wash their hands, and meticulous care should be taken in preparing bottle feeds for infants. Oral rehydration solutions should be available, or can be made up.

Exposure to sunlight

The wearing of lightweight, loose clothing, hats and sunglasses should be encouraged. High factor waterproof UVA/UVB sunblock creams should be applied several times daily.

Heat intolerance and dehydration

While resting and playing in the shade, attention should be paid to sun protection and frequent drinks, preferably of plain water, help to avoid overheating and dehydration.

Immunisation

Vaccine requirements may be different for children. Some vaccines have a higher rate of complications in children, while others do not achieve an adequate response in younger children.

Anti-malarial drugs

Children of all ages require prophylaxis in high-risk areas (Fig. 52).

Accidents

Children are accident prone. An adventurous child in an unfamiliar setting is at risk of accidents.

Bites and stings

Discourage contact with animals. Children should cover up between dusk and dawn and insect repellents and bed nets should be used. Avoid excessive amounts of DEET on small children.

Flying

Changes in cabin pressure may cause painful ears and sinuses. Swallowing and yawning may help, as may decongestants.

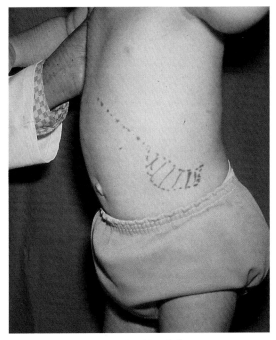

Fig. 52 Splenomegaly in a child with malaria.

Elderly travellers

Two main factors increase the risk of travel-related health problems in the elderly:
- the physiological effects of ageing on the cardiovascular, respiratory and gastrointestinal systems, and the bones and joints
- older people are more likely to suffer from chronic illnesses such as diabetes and disabilities which may limit mobility.

Health issues for elderly travellers

During air travel
- Dehydration may result from dry cabin air if fluid intake is not maintained.
- Prolonged immobilisation may predispose to thrombosis; standing and moving about in the plane may reduce this risk.
- Urinary retention may occur.
- Hypoxia can result from reduced cabin air pressure.

Potential problems
- Pre-existing medical conditions may worsen.
- There is risk of infectious diseases, especially respiratory and diarrhoeal disease. Food hygiene is essential as physiological achlorhydria predisposes to diarrhoeal disease.

Medication
- Access to medical care may be limited.
- Compartmentalised pill boxes may help (Fig. 53) with storage and compliance with medication.

Climate and topography
- Climate, especially high humidity and extremes of temperature can cause problems.
- Hypoxia at altitude may occur.
- Mobility and access may be limited.

Insurance

Comprehensive insurance is essential prior to departure.

Travel health issues for disabled travellers

Decreased mobility

Travellers with physical disabilities may find travel more difficult and stressful as a result of decreased mobility or impaired vision or hearing (Fig. 54).

Access

Access to toilet and washing facilities may be difficult.

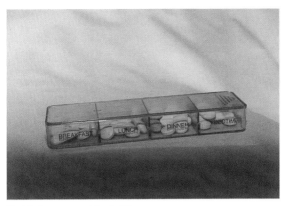

Fig. 53 Compartmentalised pill boxes.

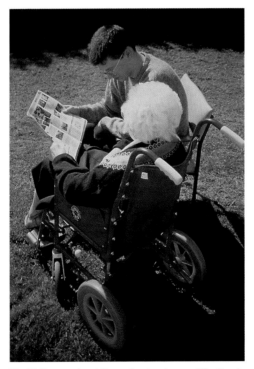

Fig. 54 Decreased mobility makes travel more difficult and stressful.

Travellers with pre-existing medical conditions

Elderly people are more likely to suffer from chronic illness but diabetes, asthma, coeliac disease and skin problems affect all ages.

Medication

- Medications may be affected by heat; insulin must not be carried in the hold of planes as it may freeze. Customs may be suspicious of drugs and syringes carried in luggage. A doctor's letter should be carried stating that the medication is prescribed for medical reasons.
- Plan in case luggage goes astray: spare medication should be carried in hand luggage.
- Comply with usual dosing schedules: diabetics need to adjust insulin dosage to cope with time zone changes.
- Interactions can occur with OTC medicines bought abroad.

Diet

- Sticking to dietary rules may be difficult where food is unfamiliar.
- It may be difficult to eat at certain times. Diabetics may need to monitor blood sugars more frequently and adjust food intake and insulin dose to take account of changes in meals and activity.

Illness while abroad

- Comprehensive insurance is required; some policies may exclude pre-existing medical conditions.
- Contingency plans in case of illness should be in place, including access to local medical care.
- A medical bracelet or medallion may alert others to medical conditions (Fig. 55).

Travellers with pre-existing psychological conditions

Such travellers may have difficulty coping with the stress of travel and with unfamiliar cultures and habits.

Coping mechanisms

- This may lead to loneliness, depression and put the traveller at risk of excessive alcohol use, the use of street drugs or inappropriate use of prescription medicines.
- In extreme cases, a traveller may harm himself/herself.

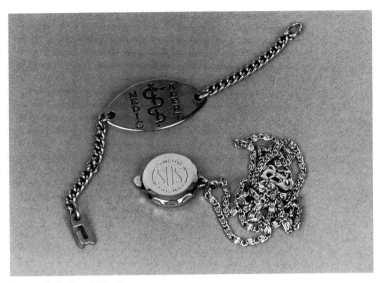

Fig. 55 Medic Alert-SOS talisman.

The HIV-positive traveller

Immune compromise may result from a number of medical conditions or organ transplantation.

HIV infection causes immune compromise, which may be severe in advanced disease. Many people with HIV travel regularly and require special advice to do so safely.

Immunisation

- Some live vaccines are contraindicated in HIV-positive individuals, especially in those who are severely immune compromised. Any vaccine may temporarily increase HIV replication so should be used only after careful evaluation of risk/benefit (Box 10).

Medication

- Medication may include regular multi-drug antiretroviral therapy, prophylactic antibiotics and emergency medication for infectious diseases.
- Medication must be taken according to schedule (Fig. 56).
- Possible interactions should be checked before using OTC drugs.
- Medication must be stored correctly and a doctor's letter provided for Customs. Some countries have entry restrictions for people with HIV.

Infectious disease

Susceptibility to infectious disease, especially diarrhoeal disease, is increased. Food and water hygiene must be strictly observed.

Disability

Previous illness and the effects of medication may have left the patient with disabilities such as peripheral neuropathy and impaired lung function, which may restrict activities.

Access to medical care

This may be difficult in remote areas and the standard of care may be lower than in the UK. Medical staff may have little or no experience of treating HIV-positive individuals. Travellers should take a brief summary of their medical condition with them.

Insurance

Read the small print; many policies do not cover HIV-positive individuals and others do not cover any illness in a person who has HIV. Some companies offer policies especially for HIV-positive travellers. Insurance should cover medical repatriation.

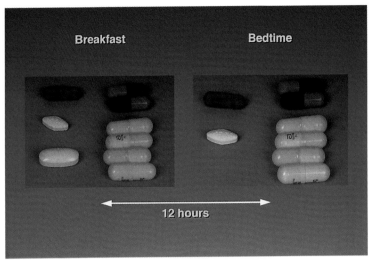

Fig. 56 HIV medication can involve complicated schedules.

Box 10 Vaccines indicated and contraindicated for HIV-positive patients as advised by the Department of Health

Indicated	Contraindicated
Measles (or MMR)	BCG
Mumps	Yellow fever
Diphtheria	Typhoid (oral)
Poliomyelitis*	
Rubella	
Hepatitis A	
Hepatitis B	
Influenza	
Meningococcus	
Pertussis	
Pneumococcal	
Rabies	
Typhoid (injection)	
Tetanus	

*Virus may be excreted for longer periods than in normal individuals; contacts should be warned to wash hands after changing a vaccinated infant's nappies. HIV-positive contacts are at greater risk than normal subjects. For symptomatic HIV-positive patients, inactivated poliomyelitis vaccine can be used at the discretion of the physician.

8 / Accidents

Introduction

Second only to cardiovascular disease in the elderly, trauma is the leading cause of mortality and morbidity in the travelling public.

Causes

Can be attributed to:
- persons
- places
- premises
- pastimes
- occupational risks.

Statistics

- All age groups are involved but unequally so.
- 19–25-year-old males are in the highest risk group.
- Accidents are not the same in different age groups.
- Road traffic accidents predominate (Fig. 57).
- Alcohol is often involved (Fig. 58).
- Drug abuse is an undocumented possibility.

Prevention

The risk factors can be identified as follows:
- Persons—lack of skill/training.
- Places—route layout, transport, terrain.
- Premises—balconies, elevators, fire escape routes, appliances.
- Pastimes—water/winter sports, mountaineering, tours (Fig. 59).
- Occupational—risks at home are carried by the traveller to host countries.

It should be noted that accident prevention is not always within the control of the ultimate victim, i.e. avalanches, uprisings or assault.

Preparation

The traveller can lessen the risk of accidents by:
- acquiring relevant skills/training
- becoming familiar with the customs of the country to be visited
- correcting personal defects, i.e. visial problems
- obeying safety guidelines, e.g. following weather reports
- limiting alcohol consumption
- being aware and wary at all times.

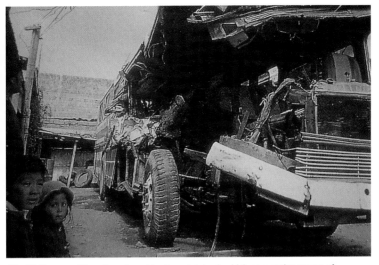

Fig. 57 Poor condition of roads and badly maintained vehicles are major causes of accidents abroad.

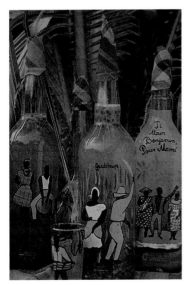

Fig. 58 Alcohol consumption is a major contributory factor to most accidents.

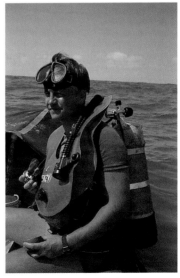

Fig. 59 Good safety standards are not guaranteed for risky pursuits.

Medical care overseas

Acute trauma is no respector of time.

Requirements

Injured persons should be transported by an experienced team, in the shortest time to a definitive care setting (Fig. 60).

Services

Travellers should note the following:
- Services can only be to the standard available in the host country.
- Tertiary care facilities may be absent.
- The closest facilities of whatever standing may be hundreds of miles away.
- Transport may be unavailable.
- Hostile terrain causes extreme difficulty for rescuers.
- Costs may not equate with those at home.
- The integrity of blood supplies cannot always be guaranteed.

Assistance

Some countries have aeromedical evacuation services:
- *Non-dedicated services*: these are provided via brokers or chartered organisations which match patient need with available transport.
- *Dedicated services*: these are less numerous than broker services.

Charges are usually higher but improved quality of care can offset the disparity in cost.

It should be noted that all such services involve the use of fixed-wing aircraft. These dedicated services are sourced from differing providers:
Sponsored by private, fee-for-service or subscription companies, e.g.:
- Med-Plane in the USA
- Vuelo de Vida in South America
- Medical Rescue International in South Africa.

Medical assistance companies acting on behalf of travel insurers, e.g.:
- Europe Assistance
- Mondial.

Charities, e.g.:
- Royal Flying Doctor Service in Australia.

Governmental agencies, e.g.:
- REGA of Switzerland.

Arising from the diversity of need and available care and costs, medical travel insurance must be a priority for travellers.

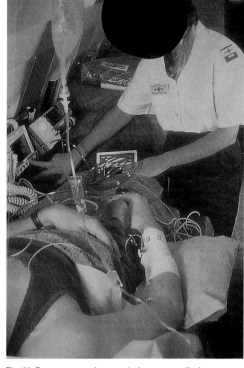

Fig. 60 Emergency assistance during aeromedical evacuation.

First aid

Definition	The first assistance given to a casualty prior to the arrival of expert care. It may involve improvisation with facilities and materials available at the time.
Aims	• To preserve life • To prevent deterioration • To promote recovery.
Other conditions and treatment	*Unconsciousness*: Place casualty in recovery position (unless neck injury is suspected) (Figs 61 & 62). *Haemorrhage*: Apply direct pressure over site and elevate (unless fracture is suspected). *Fractures*: Apply traction (along long axis in limbs) and elevate where possible after immobilisation. *Burns*: Cool down until pain ceases by whatever means available. Note: remove any constrictions before area swells but do not remove anything adhering to a burn area. *Spinal injuries*: These are best untouched until expert help arrives, but this is not always possible. A history of violent falling, bending or twisting should alert individuals to the possibility of spinal injury. Note: wounds on the forehead often accompany a spinal injury. *Shock*: Keep the head and heart low, and elevate lower limbs. Cases of electrical shock need *safe* removal from the source of injury. *Minor injuries*: Should follow the same principles but be less intense.
Personnel	Doctors and nurses do not always make the best first aid attendants.
Training	Training is readily available worldwide. In the UK, three voluntary organisations control all training courses: • St John's Ambulance • St Andrew's Ambulance Association • The British Red Cross Society. Contact telephone numbers for these organisations can be found in telephone directories and Yellow Pages.

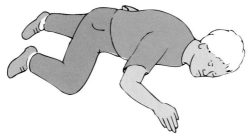

Fig. 61 Recovery position.

Open	**A** irway
Adequate	**B** reathing
Sufficient	**C** irculation

Fig. 62 ABCs of resusitation.

Traveller's diarrhoea

Clinical features

Frequent loose stools with abdominal pain and often vomiting. Fever is unusual and generally low grade. Dehydration is usually mild but may be severe. Blood can sometimes be found in the stool. Symptoms occur over usually limited period of a few days.

Aetiology

Enterotoxogenic *Escherichia coli* is most common (Fig. 63), but other causes include:
* *Shigella*
* *Salmonella*
* *Campylobacter*.

Treatment

Rehydration, but antibiotics (ciprofloxacin) early in an attack may help shorten the symptoms.

Prevention

When considering food, "boil it, cook it, peel it or forget it" is a good rule and travellers should drink boiled, purified or bottled water.

Persistent diarrhoea

Clinical features

Giardia lamblia
Symptoms develop 2–6 weeks after swallowing cysts; frequent pale, offensive bulky stools are passed. There is no blood or mucus but bloating, noisy borborygmi and flatus is common.

Diagnosis

Cysts may be found in the stool.

Clinical features

Amoebic dysentery
Diarrhoea develops gradually and may occur months after initial infections with cysts. The stools may contain blood, but unlike bacillary dysentery, fever is seldom present. Vomiting and tenesmus are uncommon.

Diagnosis

The finding of active amoebae in a fresh stool.

Complication

Amoebic liver abscesses (Fig. 64) may rupture, causing empyema, peritonitis or pericarditis, jaundice and anaemia.

Malaria (see p 39)
May present with diarrhoea and fever.

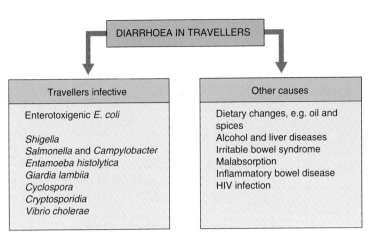

Fig. 63 Main causes of traveller's diarrhoea.

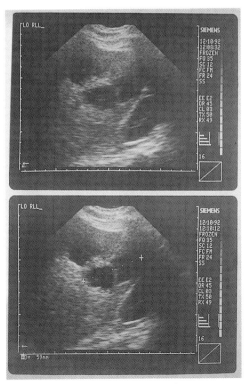

Fig. 64 CT scan of liver showing amoebic abscesses.

Respiratory disease

This is common and usually mild after exposure to unfamiliar infectious agents, but serious conditions must be considered.

Clinical features

Diphtheria
Severe sore throat. Patient is toxic with adherent membrane on palate and fauces (Fig. 65). A toxin is produced that may damage the nervous system and heart.

Diagnosis

Throat swabs should be taken from recent travellers, even if symptoms are mild.

Treatment

Penicillin and antitoxin. Prophylaxis or immunisation of contacts should be considered.

Clinical features

Legionnaires' disease
Usually pneumonia (fever, cough, shortness of breath, chest pain) but often other features such as confusion, hallucinations, dysarthria and cerebellar signs.

Diagnosis

Can be confirmed by finding immunoflorescent antigen in the urine or by serology.

Treatment

Should be empirical (until confirmed) if diagnosis is considered using erythromycin and/or rifampicin.

Clinical features

Tuberculosis and pneumocystis pneumonia
Patients present with hypoxia, minimal chest signs and diffuse shadowing on radiograph (Fig. 66). HIV infection should be considered where there are no other predisposing features.

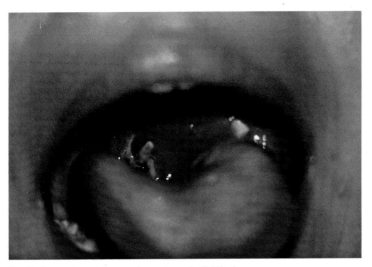

Fig. 65 Oedematous pharynx with membrane in diphtheria.

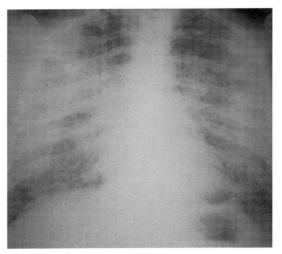

Fig. 66 Pneumocystis pneumonia can be confused with fulminant tuberculosis in those with AIDS.

Fever

Clinical features

Malaria (see p 39)
Consider in any fevered patient with suitable exposure. Fever may be irregular. Associated symptoms include diarrhoea, jaundice and confusion.

Diagnosis

Thick blood films checked by an experienced person.

Treatment

May include chloroquine or quinine but depends on type and drug resistance pattern.

Clinical features

Dengue fever
Mosquito-borne arbovirus with an incubation period of 5–8 days. Sudden onset fever, headache, severe muscular pain and often upper respiratory symptoms. Typically a maculopapular or haemorrhagic rash appears on days 3–5 (Fig. 67).

Diagnosis

Virus isolation or rising antibody titres.

Treatment

None but mortality low.

Clinical features

Viral haemorrhagic fever
Rare but high mortality, e.g. Lassa fever. Most commonly occurs in regions south of Sahara desert.

Management

Seek advice immediately; cases are managed in centralised isolation units (Fig. 68) to protect staff.
   Many other causes of fever are transmitted by insects.

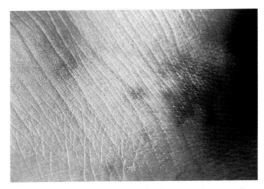

Fig. 67 A haemorrhagic rash may be due to meningococcal infection, dengue or other haemorrhagic fevers.

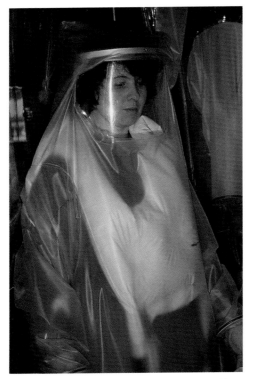

Fig. 68 Isolation for those caring for patients with highly contagious viral haemorrhagic fevers.

Rashes—with fever

Clinical features

Typhoid
Transmitted by faecal–oral route. Incubation is 1–3 weeks and most constant symptoms include fever, headache, generalised aches and pains, and anorexia. Those infected may have diarrhoea or constipation with abdominal pain. Rash is in the form of 'rose spots' on the trunk.

Diagnosis

Blood culture.

Treatment

Antibiotics, e.g. ciprofloxacin.

Clinical features

Typhus
Transmitted by arthropods such as ticks or lice; features variable but generally continuous fever, bronchitis or pneumonia. Generalised adenopathy splenomegaly. Rash is maculopapular.

Diagnosis

Clinical picture in an endemic area may be sufficient, otherwise serological tests.

Treatment

Tetracycline.

Clinical features

Lyme disease
Low-grade fever, often with headache, muscle and joint pain. Rash occurs early and is red and expanding, called 'erythema chronicum migrans' (ECM) (Fig. 69). Lyme disease is transmitted by ticks. ECM occurs at the site of the bite 3–32 days later. Late complications involve joints, cardiac and nervous system.

Treatment

Antibiotics, e.g. doxycycline.

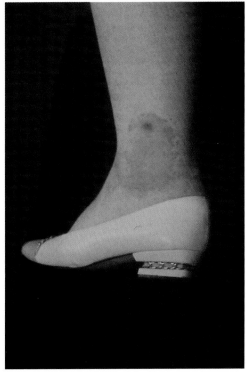

Fig. 69 Erythema chronicum migrans due to Lyme disease.

Jaundice

The commonest infective causes of jaundice are hepatitis A, B and E, and malaria. If fever is present, malaria due to haemolysis in falciparum infection must be excluded first, because of the need for urgent treatment. Once jaundice has appeared, viral hepatitis is normally afebrile (Fig. 70).

Aetiology

Hepatitis B (Fig. 71) is transmitted via blood products or sexually. Common routes of infection include sexual intercourse, I.V. drugs, tattoos, blood transfusion, or occupational exposure.

Diagnosis

Raised liver enzyme activity, IgM antibodies or hepatitis B serological markers.

Treatment

Generally supportive. Severity of acute hepatitis is related to age—children generally get milder illnesses. A rare cause of jaundice is amoebic liver abscess.

Rashes—without fever

Aetiology

Tumbu fly
Generally found in east and central Africa. Eggs are laid on clothing dried out of doors and larvae burrow into skin on contact.

Clinical features

Boil-like swelling with black dots of breathing tubes visible.

Treatment

Put Vaseline® or oil over breathing tubes and squeeze out larvae.

Prevention

Clothes dried out of doors should be ironed with a hot iron to kill eggs.

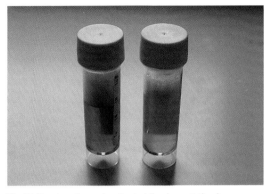

Fig. 70 Deeply yellow urine due to bile pigmentation in hepatitis A.

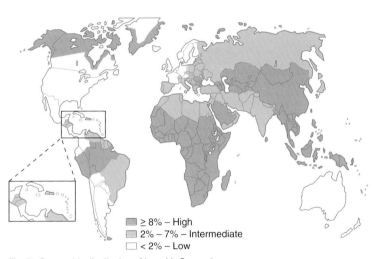

≥ 8% – High
2% – 7% – Intermediate
< 2% – Low

Fig. 71 Geographic distribution of hepatitis B prevalence.

Parasites

Clinical features

Ascaris lumbricoides (roundworm)
Eggs swallowed go through transition stages in the lungs and gut. Severe infestation may cause fever, wheeze and breathlessness during lung migration. In the gut, infestation can cause obstruction and malnutrition (Fig. 72).

Clinical features

Strongyloides stercoralis
Larvae penetrate skin; worms can multiply in the free living stage. Itchy rash (Fig. 73) at site of larval penetration, with cough, wheeze and diarrhoea. Hyperinfection may cause severe disease.

Diagnosis

Stool microscopy.

Clinical features

Cutaneous larva migrans
Hookworm larvae of an animal (usually a dog) penetrate the skin, usually the feet. A very itchy 'track-like' rash is found where the larvae migrate.

Treatment

Albendazole orally or as paste on the lesion.

Aetiology

Schistosomiasis
Adult blood flukes live in parts of the venous system. Eggs passed in urine or stools, hatch in fresh water, enter intermediate host—a water snail—then emerge as cercaria, which penetrate intact skin of the human.

Clinical features

Katayama fever: fever, urticaria, eosinophilia, diarrhoea, cough and wheeze. Later symptoms may include bloody diarrhoea or haematuria.

Late effects

Obstructive uropathy, carcinoma of bladder, kidney stones, cor pulmonale, pipestem fibrosis of liver.

Diagnosis

Urine microscopy, rectal biopsy, immunodiagnostic tests.

Treatment

Various drugs.

Aetiology

Tapeworm
Eating undercooked meat with larval stages.

Clinical features

Cause few symptoms, rarely gut obstruction.

Diagnosis

Segments of tapeworm seen in stools (Fig. 74).

Complications

Pork tapeworm may cause cysticercosis if eggs are swallowed directly. Cysts may form in muscles or subcutaneous tissues but may develop in the brain, causing epilepsy.

Treatment

Niclosamide.

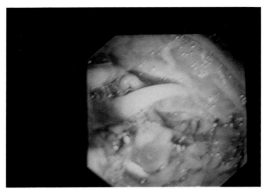

Fig. 72 *Ascaris lumbricoides* (roundworm) visualised in the stomach on endoscopy.

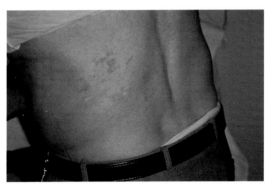

Fig. 73 Rash associated with *Strongyloides.*

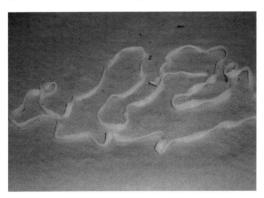

Fig. 74 Tapeworms are usually contracted through eating undercooked meats.

Introduction

Expatriate workers may be exposed to both additional health risks and multiple or severe stress. Assessment of returning expatriates requires a broad knowledge base of causes of ill health and the relational and traumatic pressures to which expatriates may be exposed.

Medical review

Candidate medical examination identifies those at unacceptable physical and mental health risk for work overseas. Medical examination on leave, by contrast, assesses the medical impact of employment abroad and emphasizes to employees their value to the agency (Fig. 75).

Medical screening should be appropriate to risk of illness. For young travellers with short terms of stay abroad, a self-administered questionnaire should identify those who need further medical evaluation. Travellers with longer terms abroad and older expatriates should be offered a full medical review. Some risk factors may only emerge during a face-to-face review. Direct questions should be asked to assess exposure to HIV, schistosomiasis (Fig. 76) and trypanosomiasis. Older, long-term expatriates who have not had access to good medical facilities deserve particular care. Altered bowel habit, angina, breast changes or signs of thyroid disorder will require appropriate investigation. Immunisations and antimalarials can be reviewed. A medical evaluation may allow identification of personal, relational, and psychological issues to be addressed.

The need for a medical review should be determined by:
• length of time stayed overseas
• particular health risks of that location
• ease of access to competent medical facilities.
A medical examination is appropriate if a traveller has:
• stayed overseas for more than 1 year
• unexplained symptoms
• returned from a particularly stressful assignment such as a war zone or refugee camp.

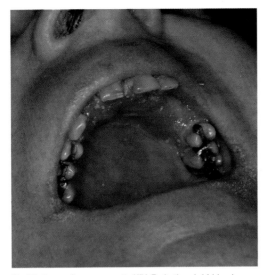

Fig. 75 Assess for exposure to HIV. Early thrush hidden by dentures in a previously undiagnosed expatriate with a presentation of CD4 count of 30/mm3.

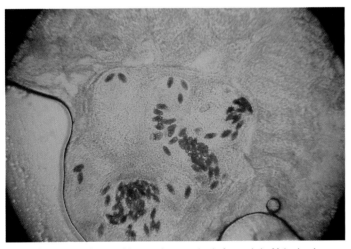

Fig. 76 *Schistosoma haematobium* ova in a rectal snip from a Lake Malawi swimmer.

Social and psychological re-adaptation for returning expatriates

Home leave

Voluntary agency policy on length of tours and home leave has altered substantially with the advent of cheap and efficient air travel. Short home leave may be treated as a fantasy time, during which there is no re-engagement with home culture. 'Reality' is left behind in the adopted country. Longer periods of home leave are important opportunities for acquiring additional skills and training, but the transitional stress of re-adapting to the parent culture is increased and may precipitate clinical depression in some individuals. In such cases, agencies should tailor home leave policy to the particular needs of the worker. Other stressors during leave may include exhausting extensive travel. Leave should be structured to include time for restoration and relaxation.

Final return — when home is no longer home

'Reverse culture shock' of final re-entry is often more difficult and re-adapting takes longer than the original move to the host country, especially for those who successfully adjusted to their new culture (Box 11). A valued job and significant role in society may have been lost. Things that once looked natural may now look extravagant and insensitive. Friends might appear unsupportive and lack understanding.

Low-grade, chronic discomfort gradually eases over a couple of years, but bereavement reactions may be severe (Fig. 77).

Serious psychological trauma

Transition is most difficult where it is unplanned and involuntary. Those evacuated due to civil war, severe illness, expulsion by a government, or failure to cope with difficult assignments may experience considerable mental pain. Guilt may be a prominent feeling for expatriates leaving national colleagues behind in situations of danger.

Post-traumatic stress disorder (PTSD) may occur following trauma, violence or rape, and agencies should make urgent arrangements for counselling, preferably on the field but otherwise immediately following an individual's return home. In some circumstances, counselling therapy outside the agency is preferable.

Box 11 A case history

A 60-year-old expatriate returned after a lifetime of service in Africa, where she had also grown up as a 'missionary kid'. She decided unwisely to make a clean break with her past, arriving with a couple of suitcases and little to remind her of her life's work. She became classically bereaved and was disturbed to find herself in tears for no apparent reason. She found it difficult to speak at public meetings where she had the opportunity to relate her life's work to others, but eventually settled more easily after a return visit to Africa.

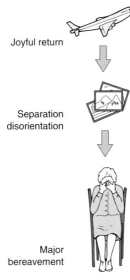

Joyful return

Separation disorientation

Major bereavement

Fig. 77 Range of individual responses after re-entry to the home country.

Re-entry and children

Children have similar transition reactions but the decision to return may not have been shared nor understood, and their parent's culture is not their own. Third-culture kids (TCKs) are defined as 'children who have spent some or all of their formative years in a culture different to that of their parents and who have therefore been reared in a unique blend of two cultures, a third culture not having a sense of belonging to either culture' (Fig. 78). An opportunity for an appropriate farewell to people and place is essential. On arrival in their parents' home country, a child may be devastated to find their previous overseas life is rejected by and incomprehensible to their new peer group.

TCKs often seem mature, with a breadth of experience of life and different cultures, but may be naive about life in the West and its sexual pressures. Younger children who have been pampered may lack basic skills such as dressing themselves or looking after their clothes and toys. TCKs' parents are often overwhelmed by their own re-entry transition difficulties and are less able to give the sensitive support that these children in transition really need. Other TCK peers or adults may play a helpful role in providing this support.

A return visit to the host country for some young people, particularly if they left in the pre-teenage phase or did not have opportunity for an appropriate farewell, may ease resettlement and enable re-assessment of their previous host country through more mature eyes. Restlessness however may continue for some years for TCKs as they search to regain a sense of belonging and later this may fuel motivation to return overseas as adults.

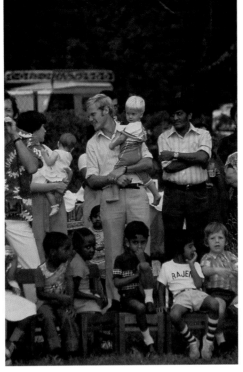

Fig. 78 'Third culture kids' at an international school in Africa, brought up in the cultural mix of Europe, Asia and Africa.

Index